BEGINNERS GUIDE

TO

CBD HEMP OIL

Experience Better Health, Faster Healing, Reduced Anxiety & Pain and Enjoy Optimum Happiness

Maurice Hauer, MD.

Contents

Title

Maurice Hauer, MD

Overview

Cannabis has remained one of the most natural, versatile and ubiquitous plants though unauthorized in many parts of the world owing to the altering effect it has on the body of a person.

Notwithstanding this mind altering effect, cannabis has provided many valuable & medicinal by products and oils including CBD hemp oil which has remedied many health challenges and ailments that would have become worse in the absence or non-existence of this natural oil.

Right from the topical application on the skin to the management of different ailments, CBD oil has myriad of health benefits. However, the original oil is not easily accessible thus hindering many persons from exploiting the benefits this natural product brings.

This book has been compiled with my 25+ years of experience in the research of Medical Marijuana and Cannabis. Thus, the major objective is to provide you with the fundamentals of CBD Hemp oil including how you can produce your own oil conveniently at the comfort of your home plus information you should know before placing an order for original

CBD oil.

So let's get started!

Chapter 1

Introduction

CBD which stands for cannabidiol belongs to the family of cannabinoid which are groups of biologically active cannabis substances that posses significant health benefits. These cannabis plants consist of myriads of chemical constituent that include enzymes, steroids, flavinoids, terpenoids and many phyto-cannabinoids.

Cannabinoids helps by modulating the body and human brain physiological systems/activities.

Hemp represent a group of high growing and extremely versatile plants which is specifically used for manufacturing thousand of industrial and commercial products varying from construction and clothing to topical ointments and oils. Only items produced from industrial hemp (< 0.3% THC) are authorized to be sold, bought, consumed and shipped. This singular property (0.3% THC) is what distinguishes "cannabis" from "hemp".

THC (tetrahydrocannabinoid) being a psychoactive component makes people feel high unlike the non-psychoactive CBD which has no inducing effect or making one feel high/'stoned'.

Mechanism of action of CBD: The Endocannabinoid System

Research on cannabis had led into the discovery of the Endocannabinoid System (ECS) which plays a major function in regulating our mood, physiology and everyday experience. This ECS can also be referred to as "the body's cannabinoid system" which consist of groups of cannabinoid receptors that are localized in the peripheral &

central nervous system and the human brain. Various researches have revealed that these receptors provide a dual communication between our body systems which can be the reason why our body system utilizes CBD. These researches have shown that CBD functions as neuro-modulator for myriad of processes such as pain sensation, appetite and motor learning among other physical and cognitive processes.

The 2 basic endocannabinoid receptors are **CB1** (located primarily in the Central and Peripheral Nervous System, brain, lungs, kidneys and Liver) and **CB2** (found primarily in the spleen and immune system). These receptors are designed specifically to work with our own natural body endocannabinoids (usually produced after exercise) and plant induced cannabinoids such as CBD and THC. The basic function of the CB2 and CB1 receptors are either to "inhibit" or "excite". This "inhibit" or "excite" process determines the way our body system including hormones will be regulated.

However, CBD does not have any direct action on the CB2 and CB1 receptors. However, they interact and facilitate other signaling systems. In other words, CBS acts indirectly by activating the signals of the body endogenous cannabinoid thus enhancing the release of the body endocannaibinoids which works on both the CB2 and CB1 receptors.

Secondly, CBD can also indirectly work on other receptors apart from cb2 and cb1 receptors. It acts on receptors such as vanilloid, adenosine and serotonin which are known to proffer antidepressant effects.

CBD being a non-psychoactive substance helps to moderate myriad effects of THC. It does this by removing THC from the CB1 receptors. Therefore, if a person is having THC intoxication, it can be remedied by administration of enough quantities of CBD oil.

Chapter 2

Types of CBD Hemp Oil

There are numerous hemp oils products available in the stores which are produced according to individual's requirements and needs. They include:

A. CBD Hemp oil Tinctures:

Do you desire fast delivery of CBD oil into the blood stream and quicker action and response? Then CBD hemp oil tinctures are highly recommended for you. These tinctures are present in wide varieties of flavors that will first freshen up your oral palate before entering the general blood circulation through the sublingual region. The significance of CBD hemp oil tinctures is thus very high and ideal especially when dealing with pain and bodily inflammation, nausea and anxiety.

B. CBD Hemp oil pure Concentrate:

This CBD isolate is composed of 99% pure CBD that has been extracted from non-GMO hemp. The oil from the hemp plant is first purified and excess waxes removed thus giving rise to a very high CBD powdered concentrates. This concentrates has no taste or smell and is very free from significant amounts of THC hence, very safe to use. Since it contains no flavor, this CBD isolate can be used through oral consumption and vaping.

C. CBD Hemp oil salves :

This type of CBD is ideal to hydrate a patchy and dry skin no matter the type of skin. Its topical application can as well be a remedy to local skin, joint discomfort and pain that may be related to musculoskeletal diseases such as fibromyalgia. Stuffed with plethora of benefits, hemp oil salves can be daily applied topically to remedy ageing, dry spots, address wrinkles and manage dryness and finally revitalize the skin cells generally.

D. CBD Hemp Oil Capsules:

Capsule is one of the commonly used CBD hemp oil commodities that are available in the local stores and market as well as among retailers. These capsules are largely patronized owing to its natural mode of ingestion. A small bottle usually contains about 30 CBD capsules. Capsules are encapsulated with minerals such as powdered turmeric or calcium which gives additional nutritional benefits as well as enhancing the flavor. Taking a capsule two times in a day is ideal to add cbd hemp oil supplements inside your meal.

E. CBD Hemp Seed Powder

If you're searching for a CBD hemp supplements that you can be putting daily in your diet then the powdered CBD hemp seed is the best choice. It is 99% pure and proffers similar benefits like the other forms of CBD hemp oil. Tender crunch and rich nutty flavor of hemp seed is delicious, convenient and provides all the nutritional advantages in a very raw form.

F. CBD Hemp oil oral applicator

An oral applicator of CBS hemp oil is extensively used sublingually to administer CBD directly into the general circulation (blood stream). This remains one of the effective and efficient ways you can consume the CBD hemp oil on a daily basis.

G. CBD Hemp oil Energy Edibles and Chews:

CBD hemp oil energy chews are available in the online market. These flavored mini chocolate bars or gummies are highly infused with CBD content. There are also minor edibles such as CBD honey and Cbd peanut butter that are composed with rich quality ingredients and can be used for snack meals or as breakfast.

H. CBD Beauty Products:

Today's markets are largely populated with beauty products and guess what? CBD is not left out. Many beauty products contain cbd hemp oil and examples of them include skin moisturizer, cleanser, skin exfoliator, night and day serum and therapeutic skin soaks.

Chapter 3

Medical/Health Benefits of CBD Hemp Oil

How to use CBD oil to Cure Various Diseases

1. Reduces Nausea and Vomiting:

CBD oil is ideal for relieving vomiting and nausea which appears as basic symptoms of various Gastrointestinal (GIT) disorders including other more serious systemic ailments. For instance, CBD

Maurice Hauer, MD

oil can be of immense help when a patient is undergoing radiotherapy or chemotherapy for various malignant tumors or cancerous cells. This implies that it can lower the chances of dreadful and uncomfortable side effect of the above stated (radiotherapy and chemotherapy) palliative measures.

2. Reduces Urge For Smoking:

Regular administration of CBD oil will enable chain smokers to quit the habit of smoking. A recent research revealed that smokers that administer CBD oil every time the urge for smoking arises smoked 30% less cigarettes than their counterparts that didn't administer the CBD oil. CBD oil can as well be a good substitute for nicotine products thus, safer with minimal side effects.

3. Prevent Tumor Growth: Myriad of studies have shown that tumors can be prevented or reduced via the use of CBD oil. Moreover, the CBD oil has been revealed to be very essential in shrinking and elimination of existing tumor cells. Also, CBD oil inhibit the development of tumor – related cancer cells thus preventing chances of developing cancerous/ malignant cells in human.

4. Pain   Relief/Anti-

Inflammatory:

Pain relief is one of the most

renowned domestic uses of

CBD oil. According to studies,

cannabinoids help in the

reduction of pain by

preventing   neuronal

transmission via the pain

pathway. It has also been

proven that CBD oil

significantly   reduces

neuropathic pain and chronic

inflammation   without

analgesic tolerance. Note: Analgesic Tolerance can often occur when you use pain medications (Analgesics) over a long period of time. However, it is not observed with CBD oil.

5. Acts as a Neuro-protective Agent:

CBD oil has natural neuro-protective property preventing neuro-degradation or suppression. It also helps in the reduction of oxidative

stress which predisposes
individuals to crohn's
diseases, gastric ulcers,
rheumatoid arthritis or
Central Nervous System
disorders such as Parkinson's
disease, multiple sclerosis or
Alzheimer's disease.

6. Reduces IBS Symptoms:
Inflammatory Bowel
Syndrome (IBS) is a syndrome
that is characterized by a
collection of distressing and
disturbing symptoms though

with no obvious physical cause. CBD oil impairs this bowel inflammation, thus relieving the individual from the underlying disturbing symptoms.

7. Skin Health:

CBD oil is one of the beneficial oil for an ideal and glowing skin. This is made possible through the inhibition of sebum production (which is the underlying cause of acne). CBD oil impairs the secretion

Maurice Hauer, MD

of sebocytes and enhances anti-proliferative effects and in the same process inhibits inflammation.

Chapter 4

Factors for Purchasing CBD Hemp Oil

6 Points to Consider while shopping for CBD Hemp Oil

1. Full spectrum CBD Oil

2. Whole plant extraction

3. Whole plant extraction process

4. Domestically grown and manufactured

5. Third party tested

6. Company transparency

1. Full spectrum CBD oil:

Full spectrum oil is oil that includes all the 80+ cannaibinoids, flavinoids, terpenes and other extra molecules that are present in the hemp plant. When you consume such full spectrum CBD oil, you will observe 100% Entourage effect (an effect that occurs when all the cannibinoids work together). That's where the magic happens because you will get

Maurice Hauer, MD

the medicinal benefits everybody is talking about. Now, we have the CBD isolate (opposite of the full spectrum CBD oil) - this refers to the CBD that's plant isolated with no other content from the hemp plant. It appears as a natural powder that's neither lab nor synthetically made. This CBD isolate has 99% purity level and the most available product that contains the highest amount of CBD. This can be added to oil and distributed in the market as CBS oil.

2. Whole plant extraction:

In addition to the full spectrum, it's important to have the oil extracted from the whole plant (i.e. the stalks, flowers and leaves) which is the most valuable part of the hemp plant. The reason for this is that a full plant extract will provide the anticipated result than one gotten from the stem or seeds. It's worthy to note that you can't extract cannaibinoids from hemp seeds. This is contrary to what is seen in various websites. Nevertheless, these seeds contain large amount of linoliec acid and omega-3-fatty acid which is the reason these seeds are used because the cannaibinoids are absorbed in the whole system better when there is fatty oil availability. But in reality, the belief that CBD or THC is extracted from hemp seed is absolutely false. There may be trace elements just because the seed is part of the plant but it's never a source of CBD hemp oil.

3. Whole plant extraction process:

The extraction process is also important. You need to ensure that the company is using a safe extraction method to remove the CBD from the hemp plant. You would want to choose a CO_2 extraction process which remains the most technological advanced procedures though it requires much expenses and expertise but it will automatically eliminate some companies from the market place. It uses extremely low temperature and high pressure to remove and preserve the oil purity. This procedure allows the extractor machine to selectively separate the cannibinoids and ultimately add the desired constituent. This remains the ultimate way THC is removed hence this procedure is considered as potent, reliable and free from chlorophyll residue. Other extraction processes are the ethanol and olive oil methods which have been explained thoroughly in the subsequent pages.

4. Domestically grown:

Another factor you should check out for is whether the CBD is domestically grown. For instance, the Kentucky supplier provides only premium whole plant CBD ingredients. They are generally grown on the US family farms and subsequently processed in the US into bulk ingredients. Furthermore, they are being produced under FDA compliance supervision and

41

facilities. These Kentucky suppliers operate with authorized license obtained from the Kentucky Department of Agriculture (DOA) which is in line with section 7606 of the US Farm bill.

The Kentucky's farmers are time tasted pioneers in hemp agriculture, agrotech and farming practices for decades (dating back to the 1700's when they began hemp farming). They are into massive teaching and training of US family farmers so that the industry can thrive even further.

Growing practices really matters as well. The Kentucky grower:

- Eliminates mold and other pathogens.

- Uses water conservation practices as well as energy conservation.

- Grows hemp in organic soil

- Etc.

5. Third Party Tested:

Another consideration is to ensure that the CBD oil is tested by a third party vendor. This is critical which is done to ensure that there are no toxins; Also, it will ensure that the CBD oil has the purity and potency being advertised. Thus, third party testing is very important so when you're shopping, ensure that you ask for third party test result so you will be sure that you're getting the correct product.

6. Company Transparency:

This is another factor to check out. The company must have high reputation with accessible support and contact address.

Transparency is important because it helps:

- eliminates cbd confusion

- build brand integrity

- boost customer's loyalty and confidence.

Chapter 5

How to Use CBD Oil

Dosages

CBD oil can be used in many distinct ways to proffer a relief to various disease conditions. It can be mixed into your drinks or foods, taken via a dropper or pipette while others can be massaged as a paste onto the skin. You can also take CBD as a capsule. Many other products appear as sprays which are designed to be taken via administration under the tongue. However there are recommended dosages for consumption that vary on various factors including individual differences, product concentration, body weight and the condition being treated. Nevertheless, It is very necessary to request for medical and professional advice while using any specific dosage.

a. Glaucoma: A dose of 20-40mg administered under the tongue is ideal to relieve eye pressure. Nevertheless, you need to be careful to avoid doses above 40mg which can intensify the pressure in the eye.

b. Schizophrenia: Take 40-1280mg CBD daily for about 4 weeks by oral administration.

c. Sleep Disorders/Insomnia: administer 40 – 160mg daily.

d. Epilepsy: Take 200-300mg of CBD daily by oral administration for a period of 5 months

e. Chronic Pain: Consume about 2.5-20mg for a maximum period of 25 days via mouth.

Side Effects of CBD Hemp Oil

Many studies have shown that a wide range of doses of CBD oil can be tolerated. No report of central nervous system disorder has been reported either heavily or slightly administered. The most notable side effects that have been observed are tiredness. Some have loss in weight, appetite and even diarrhea episodes.

Chapter 6

Legality of CBD Hemp Oil

Know Your Legal Status

Cannabis is legal for recreational or medicinal use in some of the states. Some states legalized CBD oil as a hemp product but disapproved general usage and application of medical marijuana. There are many states that have not legalized use of marijuana but posses laws that is directly related to CBD oil. Their laws vary with some states legalizing the use of CBD oil as a medication for the treatment of varieties of epileptic conditions though at a specific concentration. Below are some states in the US that have approved the use of CBD hemp oil:

Wyoming

Wisconsin

Virginia

Utah

Texas

Tennessee

South Dakota

South Carolina

Oklahoma

North Carolina

Missouri

Mississippi

Kentucky

Iowa

Indiana

Georgia

Alabama

However, each of these states has different prescription levels to posses and use the CBD hemp oil. For instance, in Missouri, an individual must show about three other alternative medications that have proven unsuccessful for the treatment of epilepsy before the administration of CBD oil.

CBD oil are increasingly popular among many

occupations, athletes and consumers alike who use it for muscle relaxation, general therapy and anxiety reduction but the legal status remains really confusing. Though it is legal to produce and distribute products with cannabis oil content within the United States. However, in some states such as Indiana, CBD is considered legal as far as it contains less than 0.3% THC which is the psychoactive compound present in cannabis. Some manufacturers violate this act and so their products are considered illegal in such cases and because of this, there has been the confiscation of CBD oil both from wholesalers and individuals.

Also, be aware that there are imported fake products mostly from Asia that contains small fraction of CBD oil. These fake products do not deliver any result and terribly mislead people. Thus, it is highly recommended that you check the composition of CBD oil before buying them. If you have CBD oil above the legal formula, it can be confiscated by the police so it is always better to order CBD oil only from trusted and reliable sellers.

Conclusion

CBD Hemp oil provides many health benefits including relieving pain/anxiety, facilitating brain co-ordination & mood relaxation and generally promotes the health and wellbeing of an individual following the presence of Omega-3 fatty acids, linoleic acid and vitamin E.

However, if you desire to treat any condition using CBD oil, ensure to contact your local healthcare providers. They will have updated information of safe and adequate CBD sources including information about the local laws that authorize usage. Furthermore, ensure that you research the laws about your state. In most of the cases, you will be required to take a particular dose.

BONUS: How to make your own CBD Hemp oil

Simple techniques (DIY)

We have 3 scientific methods for the extraction of CBD oil viz:

- Carbon (iv) oxide method
- Oil method
- Ethanol method

Maurice Hauer, MD

1. CO_2 Method:

Here, co_2 is injected into the cannabis plant at a high pressure and low temperature giving rise to the purest form of CBD oil. It is the safest and refined method for the extraction of CBD oil as it removes chlorophyll as well as other unwanted pigment and residue from the oil extract. CBD oil produced from the co_2 technique posses a very clean taste. The major limitation is that it is a very costly method.

2. Oil Method:

This is a popular method which involves the use of olive oil which serves as a carrier oil. It has started getting popularity following the added benefits of the nutrients present in the carrier oils. This oil method is a very safe method for the extraction of CBD oil as it does not produce any residue.

C. Ethanol / Alcohol Method:
CBS oil can be extracted easily
using alcohol which is a
straightforward and safe
process. An advantage this
technique has over others is
that you don't need any special
skill or expertise or equipment
to extract or produce this oil.
Thus alcohol is considered the
ideal solvent for the extraction
of cbd oil as no unpleasant or
harmful residue is
encountered thus it's highly

suitable for consumption /usage.

Materials/ Ingredients

1. Cannabis buds (30g)

2. Alcohol (4 litres)

3. Glass or ceramic bowl

4. Sieve

5. Double boiler

6. Catchment container

7. Plastic syringe

8. Wooden spoon

9. Silicon spatula.

Procedure:

Maurice Hauer, MD

1. The first and foremost step involves soaking the cannabis plant material in a bowl containing cold alcohol for about 5 minutes.

2. Stir with a plastic spoon for 3 minutes and then sieve this mixture into a separate bowl.

3. Using a coffee filter, sieve the mixture and distill the liquid till the volume of the alcohol becomes reduced to about 80% (Note: Do this outside if you are using hot

plate or rice cooker to evaporate the alcohol because the fumes are flammable)

4. Next, pour the liquid remaining into a separate small bowl and heat on a coffee machine hot plate for a period of 24 hours. The aim is to remove any other alcohol remaining in the bowl.

5. The last step involves checking if alcohol is still remaining. You can do this by dipping a paperclip into the oil

and lighten with a match. If you notice any spark, alcohol is still present thus, it should be dried further on the coffee machine for extra hours.

6. You can now store your oil if desired. Using a medical syringe, draw the oil into it and store it in the fridge.

Advantages of producing your own oil

1. You determine the quality of your product as well as choose

your choice strain based on your desire.

2. You can produce a product that can be used for local situations or consumed for some internal medical conditions.

3. You can produce your CBD oil at a relatively low cost.

4. You can either omit or add the ingredients accordingly based on your choice.

About The Author

Dr Maurice Hauer is a seasoned pathologist and an expert in medical marijuana and cannabis having been in the profession for decades. He has many papers and publications to his credit including **"The Health Benefits of Cannabis: Anti-inflammatory and Analgesic properties"** among many others.

He resides in Indiana with his family and currently carrying out further research on CBD oil

For your questions or comments, kindly contact me via email: Bestauthor02@gmail.com and I will reply immediately.

Made in the USA
Lexington, KY
29 May 2018